HOW DO I START STRENGTH TRAINING OR RESISTANCE TRAINING

HOW DO I START STRENGTH TRAINING OR RESISTANCE TRAINING

A.D RAMS

Contents

CHAPTER ONE

INTRODUCTION

Starting a strength training or resistance training program is a big step in enhancing your general health and fitness. Strength training may be very beneficial for all fitness levels, including beginners and those making a comeback to fitness. Some of the benefits include greater muscle strength, improved bone density, metabolism, and functional fitness for daily tasks.

Through the use of resistance, strength training encourages your muscles to adapt and get stronger over time. This type of exercise includes a range of methods, such as bodyweight exercises, lifting weights, using resistance bands, and using gym equipment. Strength and fitness can be continuously improved by gradually raising the resistance or intensity of your workouts, which will keep your muscles challenged.

We'll go over the foundations of beginning strength training or resistance training in this book, which includes important ideas, necessary tools, considerations for your workout, and beginner-friendly advice. Strength training is a flexible and efficient way to reach your goals, whether they be to gain muscle, increase athletic performance, or just improve your general health and fitness.

Come along as we explore the realm of strength training and learn how to begin your path to being a better, more fit, and healthier version of yourself.

Strength training is essential for general fitness and well-being.

With so many advantages for general health and fitness, strength training is a vital part of a comprehensive fitness program. Strength training is essential for the following main reasons:

Enhanced Muscle Strength and Endurance: Resistance training works your muscles in a demanding manner, which increases your muscles' strength and endurance. Your muscles will eventually adjust to the demands of resistance training, making you stronger and better able to carry out daily duties.

Better Body Composition: Strength training can help you lose body fat and gain lean muscle mass, which will enhance your body composition. Strength training supports weight management and fat loss efforts by improving calorie burning during and after exercises by boosting muscle mass and metabolism.

Improved Bone Health: By increasing bone density and stimulating bone remodeling, weight-bearing and resistance training lower the risk of osteoporosis and fractures. Maintaining bone health is notably benefited by strength training, especially when bone density gradually decreases with age.

Enhanced Metabolic Rate: Even while at rest, muscle tissue burns calories since it has an active metabolism. Gaining more muscle mass through strength training will increase your metabolic rate and improve your overall energy expenditure, which will help you reach and stay at a healthy weight.

Strengthening the muscles, tendons, and ligaments surrounding the joints improves joint stability and lowers the chance of injury. This leads to an improvement in joint health and function. Greater muscle mass contributes to improved joint health, flexibility, and mobility by supporting the joints more effectively.

Enhanced Functional Fitness: Your capacity to carry out daily tasks with ease and efficiency is referred to as functional fitness, and strength training enhances it. Strength training improves functional ability and lowers the risk of injury during daily tasks by strengthening muscles used in frequent movements like bending, lifting, and reaching.

Improved Posture and Balance: Strength training activities work the stabilizing and core muscles, which improve alignment, balance, and posture. In addition to improving one's physical attractiveness, good posture lowers the chance of back discomfort and musculoskeletal problems.

Enhanced Sports Performance: By increasing muscle strength, power, speed, agility, and endurance, strength training can boost sports performance. Strength training is a component of training regimens for athletes in a variety of sports, as it gives them a competitive advantage and lowers their risk of injury during competition.

Decreased Risk of Chronic Illness: Consistent strength training has been linked to a lower risk of long-term illnesses like diabetes, heart disease, and several forms of cancer. Strength training increases insulin sensitivity, metabolic efficiency, and cardiovascular health, all of which promote long life and the prevention of disease.

Strength training has been found to have a good impact on mental health and well-being.

Specifically, it has been shown to reduce feelings of stress, anxiety, and depression. Exercise triggers the production of endorphins, which are happy-making and calming neurotransmitters that enhance mood and cognitive performance.

All things considered, adding strength training to your exercise regimen has several advantages for your physical and emotional well-being. Strength training offers a flexible and efficient way to reach your health and fitness objectives, whether they be to increase muscle mass, reduce body fat, boost athletic performance, or just improve your general well-being.

Recognizing Strength Training's Advantages

Resistance training, commonly referred to as strength training, has several advantages for general health and fitness. Here's a closer look at the benefits of strength training:

Enhanced muscular Strength and Endurance: Strength training increases muscular strength and endurance by subjecting the muscles to repeated contractions against resistance. Your muscles adapt by growing stronger and more resilient as you gradually overwork them, making it easier and more efficient for you to carry out daily tasks.

Better Body Composition: Strength training contributes to a decrease in body fat percentage and an increase in lean muscle mass, improving body composition. A higher ratio of muscle to fat will give you a more defined and toned body. Furthermore, muscular tissue contributes to weight control and fat loss efforts since it is metabolically active, burning more calories at rest than fat tissue.

Improved Bone Health: By increasing bone density and stimulating bone remodeling, weight-bearing and resistance training lower the risk of osteoporosis and fractures. Maintaining bone health is notably benefited by strength training, especially when bone density gradually decreases with age.

Enhanced Metabolism: Even when at rest, muscle tissue burns calories since it is metabolically active. Your basal metabolic rate (BMR) can be raised via strength training to build muscle mass, which will increase your daily calorie expenditure. It may be simpler to maintain a healthy weight and help with weight management attempts.

Strengthening the muscles, tendons, and ligaments surrounding the joints improves joint stability and lowers the chance of injury. This leads to an improvement in joint health and function. Greater muscle mass contributes to improved joint health, flexibility, and mobility by supporting the joints more effectively. This might be especially helpful for people who have joint pain or arthritis.

Enhanced Functional Fitness: Your capacity to carry out everyday tasks with comfort and effectiveness is referred to as functional fitness.

Strength training strengthens the muscles used in everyday motions such as bending, lifting, and reaching, hence increasing functional capability. You'll improve your capacity to carry out daily duties and lower your chance of injury by strengthening these muscles.

Improved Posture and Balance: Strength training activities work the stabilizing and core muscles, which improve alignment, balance, and posture. In addition to improving one's physical attractiveness, good posture lowers the chance of back discomfort and musculoskeletal problems. Improved balance can also lower the chance of falling, particularly for elderly persons.

Enhanced Metabolic Health: Insulin sensitivity, blood sugar regulation, and cholesterol profile are just a few of the metabolic health benefits that come with strength training. Frequent strength training can improve general health and longevity by lowering the risk of metabolic diseases including type 2 diabetes and metabolic syndrome.

Improved Mental Health and Well-Being: Research has demonstrated that strength training improves mental health and well-being by reducing stress, anxiety, and depressive symptoms, among other things. Exercise triggers the production of endorphins, which are happy-making and calming neurotransmitters that enhance mood and cognitive performance.

Decreased Risk of Chronic Illness: Consistent strength training has been linked to a lower risk of long-term illnesses like heart disease, stroke, high blood pressure, and several cancers.

CHAPTER TWO

Strength training increases longevity and prevents disease by lowering blood pressure, reducing inflammation, and improving cardiovascular health.

Numerous advantages of strength training exist for general health and fitness, such as better bone health, increased metabolism, improved joint health and function, better posture and balance, improved metabolic health, improved mental health and well-being, and a lower risk of chronic disease. Strength training also improves muscle strength and endurance. Strength training can enhance your quality of life while assisting you in reaching your fitness and health objectives.

Setting Objectives and Evaluating Preparedness

To guarantee a safe and successful training experience, it's critical to evaluate your preparation and set realistic goals prior to beginning a strength training or resistance training program. To evaluate your preparedness and set objectives before beginning strength training, follow these steps:

Health Assessment: It's important to evaluate your present state of health before starting any new workout regimen. Take into account things like any current health issues, injuries, or physical restrictions that can limit your capacity to engage in strength training. To be sure strength training is safe and suitable for your particular needs and health state, speak with a healthcare professional, such as your doctor or a certified personal trainer.

Fitness Assessment: Determine where you are at in terms of fitness before beginning strength training. Examine your physical attributes, including your flexibility, muscular strength, cardiovascular endurance, and muscular strength. To determine your current fitness level and areas for growth, do some simple exercises like planks, push-ups, squats, and flexibility drills.

Establish Objectives: Clearly state your intentions before beginning strength training. Think about your goals for strength training: boosting functional fitness, lowering your chance of injury, improving body composition, or growing muscle strength and mass. Throughout your training process, setting SMART (specific, measurable, achievable, relevant, and time-bound) goals will help you stay motivated and focused.

Think About Personal Preferences: When establishing strength training objectives, take into account your hobbies, preferences, and lifestyle choices. Think about things like your desired workout location (gym, home), your availability of time, your ability to obtain equipment, and your favorite type of exercise (bodyweight exercises, resistance bands, free weights, etc.). Select training modes and routines that you will find enjoyable and likely to maintain over time.

Start cautiously and Increase Gradually: In order to prevent injury and overtraining, it's critical to begin strength training cautiously and increase it gradually if you're new to it. Start off with smaller weights and fewer repetitions, paying close attention to developing good form and technique for each exercise. As your strength and conditioning improve over time, gradually increase the volume, complexity, and intensity of your workouts.

Create a Training Schedule: Based on your objectives, availability, and personal preferences, decide how frequently you will perform strength training sessions. Try to do strength training two or three days a week, with rest days in between to allow for recuperation. Establish a consistent workout routine that you can realistically stick to for the duration of the program because consistency is essential.

Track Your Development: Observe your advancements and changes throughout time. Maintain a training log or utilize a fitness monitoring application to document your workouts, including exercises, repetitions, sets, weights, and any additional pertinent information. Monitoring your development gives you encouragement to keep working toward your objectives by enabling you to see how far you've come.

You can successfully begin strength training and position yourself to succeed in reaching your fitness objectives by evaluating your preparation, defining specific goals, taking into account personal preferences, starting cautiously, creating a training regimen, and monitoring your progress. While you continue on your strength training adventure, keep in mind to pay attention to your body, focus correct form and technique, and challenge yourself progressively. Consider working with a qualified personal trainer who can offer individualized training and support catered to your unique needs and goals if you're not sure where to start or need direction.

Acquiring Fundamental Exercise Concepts

Starting a strength training or resistance training program that is both safe and successful requires familiarity with fundamental exercise principles. Gaining an understanding of these concepts will enable you to execute workouts correctly, reduce your chance of injury, and optimize your performance. Before beginning strength training, familiarize yourself with the following basic exercise principles:

Correct Form and Technique: For exercises to be performed safely and efficiently, proper form and technique are essential. Prioritize perfecting the form for every exercise before boosting the weight or intensity. It is important to pay attention to joint alignment, movement patterns, and body alignment in order to promote appropriate muscle engagement and lower the chance of injury.

Progressive Overload: To keep pushing your muscles and encouraging growth, progressive overload is the idea of progressively increasing the volume, resistance, or intensity of your workouts over time. This can be accomplished by working with heavier weights, doing more sets or repetitions, or cutting short the rest intervals in between sets. You can guarantee that your muscles continue to adapt and enhance your strength and fitness by gradually increasing the demands placed on them.

Muscle Symmetry and Balance: Preventing imbalances and lowering the risk of injury need symmetry and balance between opposing muscle groups. To encourage muscular balance and symmetry, include workouts that work both the agonist (primary) and antagonist (opposing) muscle groups. For example, to preserve upper body balance, pair workouts that engage the chest (push-ups) with activities that work the back (rows).

Full Range of Motion: To enhance joint mobility, optimize muscle activation and flexibility, and lower the risk of injury, carry out exercises across their whole range of motion. Repetitions should not be shortened or compromised by employing momentum or an insufficient range of motion. Maintain control throughout the whole range of movements while emphasizing quality above quantity.

Rest and Recovery: Give yourself enough time to relax and recuperate in between sessions so that your muscles can rebuild and strengthen. Fatigue, a decline in performance, and an elevated risk of injury can result from overtraining. To encourage healing and avoid overuse injuries, plan rest or active recovery days in between strength training sessions.

Variety and Progression: To target different muscle groups and avoid boredom, mix up your strength training routine using a range of exercises and training techniques. By varying your regimen, adding new exercises, or experimenting with new equipment, you may gradually push yourself. Exercise routines are kept engaging and encourage ongoing gains in strength and fitness with variety and progression.

Warm-Up and Cool-Down: To get your body ready for activity and speed up recovery, make sure your strength training regimen always includes a warm-up and cool-down. A dynamic warm-up, which includes dynamic stretching and light exercise, boosts body temperature, improves blood flow, and gets muscles ready for action. Static stretching and foam rolling as part of a cool-down assist ease pain in the muscles, increase flexibility, and encourage relaxation.

Listen to Your Body: During exercise, pay attention to the signals from your body and modify your workouts as necessary. In order to prevent injury, adjust the workout or lower the intensity if you feel pain, discomfort, or exhaustion. It's important to push oneself, but never at the price of technique or safety.

You can start a strength training or resistance training program that is safe, efficient, and satisfying by understanding and putting these fundamental exercise principles into practice. Prioritize good form and technique, gradually increase the intensity of your workouts, keep your balance and symmetry, provide enough time for rest and recuperation, add diversity and progression, implement warm-up and cool-down routines, and pay attention to your body's signals. You may attain your health and fitness objectives and increase your strength and fitness level with perseverance and commitment.

Initially, bodyweight exercises

If you are new to exercising or have limited access to equipment, bodyweight exercises are a great way to start your strength or resistance training adventure. Anybody can perform bodyweight exercises, which are accessible and convenient since they only require your own body weight as resistance, to increase muscular tone and build strength. The following is how to begin bodyweight exercises:

Learn the Fundamentals: Start with basic bodyweight exercises that focus on the main muscle groups and movement patterns. These consist of movements including planks, bodyweight rows, push-ups, pull-ups (or modified versions), squats, and lunges. Prioritize perfecting form and technique for every exercise before moving on to increasingly complex versions.

Start Slowly and Increase Gradually: If you're not familiar with strength training or exercise, begin each exercise with a reasonable amount of repetitions and sets. For every exercise, aim for one to three sets of eight to twelve repetitions, emphasizing quality above number. To keep your muscles challenged, progressively up the amount of repetitions, sets, or complexity of the exercises as you gain confidence in them and your strength increases.

Exercise range: To target different muscle groups and movement patterns, mix up your practice with a range of bodyweight exercises. This promotes muscular growth, keeps workouts interesting, and guarantees a complete exercise. To achieve balanced workouts, mix and match exercises for your core, lower body, and upper body.

Emphasis on Form and Technique: To maximize the benefits of bodyweight exercises and lower the risk of injury, proper form and technique are crucial. During each exercise, pay special attention to joint placement, body alignment, and movement patterns. Maintain neutral spine posture, contract your core muscles, and go through the entire range of motion with deliberate control.

Adapt as Needed: Don't be scared to change up bodyweight exercises to fit your skills and fitness level. If an exercise seems too difficult, try an adapted version or get assistance with the movement from a chair or wall. For instance, you can use a resistance band to help with aided pull-ups or substitute complete push-ups with knee push-ups.

Advance Over Time: To keep your muscles challenged as you get stronger and more adept at bodyweight exercises, progressively move on to more complex variations or up the difficulty of the exercises. You can advance by trying more difficult exercise variations (such pistol squats and handstand push-ups), extending the amount of repetitions or sets, or adding resistance (like utilizing a backpack filled with books for extra weight).

Listen to Your Body: During exercise, pay attention to your body's input and modify your exercises as necessary. If you feel tired, in pain, or uncomfortable, stop and take a break or lessen the intensity of the workout. It's important to push oneself, but never at the price of technique or safety.

Incorporate a Warm-Up and Cool-Down: To get your body ready for exercise and lower your chance of injury, warm up dynamically before beginning any workout. Incorporate physical activities like stationary jogging, arm circles, leg swings, and dynamic stretches to promote blood circulation and facilitate muscular elasticity. Complete your workout with a static stretch cool-down to increase your flexibility and encourage relaxation.

By beginning with bodyweight exercises and according to these guidelines, you can enhance muscle tone, develop strength, and create a strong basis for future advancements in your strength training or resistance training endeavors. Always start out cautiously, pay attention to form, pay attention to your body, and make incremental growth over time. Your strength, endurance, and general fitness will all increase with perseverance and commitment.

Overview of Tools and Equipment

Having the proper tools and equipment when beginning strength or resistance training is crucial to the success of your workouts. For those just starting out, the following equipment and tools are essential:

Bodyweight Exercises: Since they don't require a lot of equipment and can be done anywhere, bodyweight exercises are a great place for beginners to start. Planks, squats, lunges, push-ups, and bodyweight rows are a few bodyweight exercises. These workouts enhance functional fitness and strengthen the fundamental muscles.

Dumbbells: Dumbbells are useful and efficient strength training equipment that let you work out at different intensities and target different muscle areas. Dumbbells of mild to moderate weight are a good place for beginners to start, and as they gain strength, they can progressively raise the weight. Exercises using dumbbells include goblet squats, shoulder presses, chest presses, and bicep curls.

Resistance bands are a cost-effective, lightweight, and adaptable training aid for resistance exercise. All fitness levels can use them since they offer varied resistance throughout the range of action. Exercises like leg presses, sitting rows, lateral raises, and bicep curls can all be done using resistance bands.

Kettlebells: Another fantastic tool for strength training, kettlebells have special advantages such improved grip strength, stability, and cardiovascular conditioning. Kettlebell swings, goblet squats, Turkish get-ups, and kettlebell rows are among the exercises that beginners can perform with a moderate-weight kettlebell.

Barbells: When performing compound workouts that work many muscular groups at once, barbells are frequently used. Before moving on to higher weights, beginners can begin with smaller barbells or training bars to ensure appropriate form. Barbells can be used for exercises including bent-over rows, bench presses, squats, and deadlifts.

Weight Bench: A weight bench offers a steady platform on which to execute a range of exercises, such as seated rows, shoulder presses, and chest presses. Novices can begin with a flat bench and work their way up to incline or decline varieties. Exercises like tricep dips, step-ups, and reverse crunches can also be performed on a weight bench.

Stability Ball: Often referred to as an exercise ball or Swiss ball, a stability ball can provide some instability to your exercises, which will strengthen your core and enhance your balance and coordination. A stability ball can be used by beginners for workouts including wall squats, hamstring curls, crunches, and push-ups.

Mat: A fitness mat improves comfort and lowers the chance of injury by offering support and padding for stretches and floor workouts. For exercises like planks, mountain climbers, Russian twists, and yoga-inspired positions, beginners can utilize a mat.

Pull-Up Bar: A pull-up bar is an easy-to-use but powerful tool for building upper body strength, especially in the arms, shoulders, and back. Exercises like chin-ups, hanging leg lifts, and pull-ups can be performed by beginners using a pull-up bar. While some pull-up bars are freestanding or fasten to a power rack, others can be fixed to a door frame.

Timer or stopwatch: You can use a timer or stopwatch to keep track of the amount of time you spend working out, to time intervals for circuit training, or to record the rest times in between sets. This makes sure you're exercising effectively and get closer to your fitness objectives.

All of the main muscle groups can be targeted and overall strength and fitness can be enhanced by including these necessary tools and equipment into your strength training or resistance training regimen. To minimize injuries and achieve the best possible outcomes, always start with lower weights or resistance levels and concentrate on correct form and technique. To keep moving closer to your fitness objectives, progressively up the difficulty and intensity of your workouts as you acquire confidence and experience.

Creating Your Initial Strength Training Program

As you start your fitness journey, creating your first strength training regimen may be a fun and inspiring experience. This is a step-by-step approach to assist you in developing a beginner-friendly, well-rounded strength training program:

Prior to creating your routine, make sure your fitness objectives are clear. Are you trying to get stronger, gain more muscle, increase endurance, or get fitter overall? Having clear goals will help you tailor your routine to meet your specific needs and objectives.

Exercise Selection: Include a range of isolation and compound exercises in your program that focus on the main muscle groups.

Exercises that target specific muscles are called isolation workouts, whereas compound exercises train multiple muscle groups at once. Squats, deadlifts, bench presses, and rows are a few examples of complicated workouts; bicep curls, tricep extensions, and lateral raises are examples of isolation exercises.

Establish Frequency: Considering your timetable, objectives, and recuperation requirements, choose how frequently you will strength train each week. Beginners usually get the most out of exercising two to three times a week, interspersed with at least one day off to promote muscle growth and healing.

Sets and Repetitions: For beginning exercisers, try to complete 2-3 sets of each exercise, completing 8–12 repetitions in each set. While allowing for correct form and technique, this rep range is perfect for increasing muscle endurance and strength. As you gain strength, progressively increase the weight until you can perform the appropriate number of repetitions with proper form.

Plan Your Workout Split: Choose the way you'll split up your workouts between training sessions. Beginners often use a full-body training regimen that hits all of the major muscle groups throughout each session. As an alternative, you can divide your workouts into groupings of muscles (upper body, lower body) or types of action (legs, push, pull, etc.).

Include a Warm-Up and Cool-Down: To get your muscles and joints ready for exercise, boost blood flow, and lower your chance of injury, start every workout with a vigorous warm-up. Include dynamic exercises like bodyweight squats, hip circles, leg swings, and arm swings. Use static stretches to increase flexibility and encourage relaxation after your workout.

Progression: To keep pushing your muscles and encouraging strength gains, gradually up the intensity of your workouts over time. This can be achieved by adding more difficult exercise variations to your routine as you get stronger and more skilled, or by increasing the weight, repetitions, or sets of your current exercises.

Rest and Recovery: To help your muscles heal and get stronger, give yourself enough time to relax and recuperate in between workouts and sets. To promote recovery and muscular growth, aim for 1-2 minutes of rest in between sets and make sure you receive enough sleep every night.

Example of a Beginner's Full-Body Strength Training Program:

3 sets of 10 repetitions for squats

3 sets of 10 reps for push-ups

3 sets of 10 repetitions for bent-over rows

Bench Press using Dumbbells: Three Sets x Ten Reps

Deadlifts: 3 sets of 10 repetitions

Reps for Bicep Curls: 3 sets of 10

Trenches Dips: 3 sets of 10 repetitions

Plank: three 30-second sets

Never forget to begin your exercises with smaller weights and concentrate on perfecting form and technique before stepping up the intensity. Pay attention to your body; if you feel pain or discomfort, stop exercising and get advice from a healthcare physician or fitness expert. Over time, strength, muscular tone, and general fitness will all improve with regularity, commitment, and increasing overload.

Creating a Reliable Schedule

A strength training or resistance training regimen must be started and maintained with a regular schedule. To make a schedule that suits you, follow these steps:

Determine Your Availability: To begin, look over your weekly schedule and find any gaps in which you can perform strength training. Take into account elements like obligations to your family, your job, your social life, and other commitments. Choose the days and hours that you can actually dedicate to your workout regimen without being overly anxious or agitated.

Make consistency a priority: Strength training progresses only when consistency is maintained. To see benefits and keep up momentum, try to work out two or three times a week at minimum. Select a timetable that will enable you to train consistently with little breaks or time between sessions. Long-term motivation, strength, and positive habits can all be developed with consistent training.

Choose Your Training Days: Depending on your tastes and availability, choose the days of the week you'll commit to strength training. While some people prefer to space out their workouts throughout the week, others prefer to train on consecutive days. Select a timetable that fits your lifestyle and provides enough time for relaxation and recuperation in between sessions.

CHAPTER THREE

Plan Around Other Activities: To maintain flexibility and balance, schedule your strength training around other activities in your life. Plan your workouts taking into account things like job schedules, social obligations, and leisure activities. Regarding what you can fit into your schedule, be practical and adapt as necessary.

Establish Workout Times: Schedule your strength training sessions in advance and see them as commitments that you cannot skip.

Whether you are an early riser, an afternoon or an evening trainer, pick a time that best suits your energy levels and fits into your daily schedule. Timing your workouts consistently will help you form a habit and find it simpler to keep to your program.

Set Up Your Environment: Make sure your strength training space is comfortable to increase your chances of success. Set up your exercise area with the required weights and implements, including a mat, resistance bands, and dumbbells. Make it as simple as possible to begin your training session by removing any hurdles or distractions that could cause it to go off course.

Be Adaptable and Flexible: Unexpected events might occur in life, so you might need to modify your training plan at times to account for altered routines or other adjustments. Be adaptive and flexible, and don't be too hard on yourself if you have to reschedule or miss a session. The secret is to quickly get back on track and maintain your dedication to your fitness objectives.

Monitor Your Progress: To stay accountable and inspired, keep a record of your workouts and advancement. Keep track of workout specifics including exercises, sets, reps, weights, and any notes or observations in a fitness notebook, workout app, or spreadsheet. Monitoring your development gives you encouragement to keep going forward by letting you see how far you've come.

You'll position yourself for success in reaching your fitness objectives by making frequent exercises a priority and creating a consistent program for strength training. Remind yourself to be kind to yourself, stick to your regimen, and acknowledge your accomplishments as you go. You will eventually gain strength, increase your level of fitness, and reap the many advantages of strength training if you put in the necessary time and effort.

Advice on Moving Forward and Overcoming Obstacles

Progress and conquering obstacles are essential components of any strength or resistance training program. The following advice can help you advance successfully and get beyond typical obstacles:

Increase Intensity Gradually: The secret to improving your strength training is progressive overload. By using greater weights, completing more sets or repetitions, or cutting short the rest intervals in between sets, you can gradually raise the intensity of your workouts. Try to gradually increase the amount of work you put into your muscles to encourage growth and adaptation.

Focus on Form and Technique: To minimize the chance of injury and optimize outcomes, place a high priority on using appropriate form and technique during your workouts. When lifting larger weights, be mindful of your body alignment, joint placement, and movement patterns. Do not use momentum or compensating motions. Exercise number is not as crucial as quality of movement, so concentrate on performing each exercise with control and accuracy.

Change Up Your Routine: By adding variation to your routine, you can keep your workouts interesting and exciting. To target different muscle groups and movement patterns, try experimenting with different exercises, training modalities, and workout styles. This keeps things interesting, encourages muscular growth, and keeps performance and strength plateaus at bay.

Establish Realistic Goals: To help you stay motivated and guide your development, set SMART (specific, measurable, realistic, relevant, and time-bound) goals. Divide more ambitious objectives into more doable benchmarks, and acknowledge and appreciate your progress along the way. As your situation and progress warrant it, revise your objectives.

Listen to Your Body: As you exercise, pay attention to the cues your body gives you, and adjust your routines accordingly. Reduce the intensity of your workout or quit if you're feeling exhausted, in pain, or uncomfortable. Pushing oneself is vital, but never at the expense of safety or technique. Recognize your limitations and refrain from overexerting yourself, particularly when you're healing from a disease or accident.

Prioritize Recovery: To maximize recovery and avoid overtraining, allot enough time for rest and recuperation in between sessions. To promote muscle growth and recovery, include rest days in your training plan and provide adequate attention to sleep, nutrition, hydration, and stress management. Pay attention to your body's need for recuperation and relaxation, and don't be afraid to schedule more days off if necessary.

Seek Professional Advice: To assist you in creating a customized training plan, learning correct technique, and receiving direction and support along the way, think about working with a qualified personal trainer or strength coach. A competent expert may offer insightful criticism, responsibility, and inspiration to support you in accomplishing your objectives in a safe and efficient manner.

Remain Consistent: Strength training advancement requires consistency. Adhere to your exercise regimen, even on the days when you're not feeling inspired or driven. Remind yourself that improvement requires time and work, and despite obstacles or disappointments, remain dedicated to your fitness objectives. No matter how tiny your accomplishments may seem, acknowledge them and keep pushing forward with tenacity and resolve.

By adding these pointers to your strength training or resistance training regimen, you'll be able to overcome obstacles, make steady progress, and eventually reach your fitness objectives. Always remember to appreciate the process of self-improvement and growth, have patience with yourself, and remain goal-focused.

Including Exercises for Warm-Up and Cool-Down

It's imperative to include warm-up and cool-down exercises to prime your body for strength or resistance training and to facilitate post-exercise recovery. The following are some tips for including warm-up and cool-down exercises into your workouts:

Warm-up:

Dynamic exercises: To enhance blood flow to your muscles and elevate your heart rate, begin your warm-up with dynamic exercises. Arm circles, leg swings, shoulder rotations, hip circles, and stationary jogging are a few examples.

Mobility Exercises: To increase joint flexibility and mobility, engage in mobility exercises. Use exercises that target specific body parts used in strength training, such as arm circles, leg swings, torso twists, and hip hinges.

Activation Exercises: Prior to working out, use activation exercises to target and activate particular muscle groups. These workouts enhance muscle recruitment during strength training activities and help prepare your muscles for action. Scapular retractions, band walks, glute bridges, and bodyweight squats are a few examples.

Sport-Specific Movements: Incorporate sport-specific movements into your warm-up routine if you're doing a particular kind of strength or resistance training. To warm up your lower body muscles for an exercise like squats, for instance, try doing leg swings or bodyweight squats.

Gradual Progression: Raise the intensity of your warm-up gradually to correspond with the demands of your exercise. As your body temperature rises and your muscles become more prepared for activity, start with easier motions and work your way up to more dynamic and difficult activities.

Chill Out:

Static Stretching: To increase flexibility and relieve muscle tension, perform static stretching exercises following your strength or resistance training session. Stretching should be concentrated on the main muscular groups that you utilized during your workout. Hold each stretch for 15 to 30 seconds, then take deep breaths to let the muscles relax.

Foam Rolling: Apply self-myofascial release (SMR) techniques to tense or aching muscles with a foam roller or massage tool. By dissolving adhesions and knots in the muscle tissue, foam rolling eases discomfort and speeds up healing. Roll each muscle group for one to two minutes, paying particular attention to any soreness or tightness.

Deep Breathing and Relaxation: To assist your body in entering a condition of rest and recuperation, spend a few minutes practicing deep breathing and relaxation techniques. Shut your eyes, concentrate on your breathing, and let your body unwind as you let go of any stress or strain that has built up from your workout.

Nutrition and Hydration: After working out, drink some water to replenish the fluids your body lost through perspiration. Eat a well-balanced lunch or snack with protein and carbohydrates after working out to aid in muscle regeneration and restore glycogen storage.

Think and Make a Plan: Give your workout some thought, as well as your post-workout emotions. Make a note of any discomfort or areas that you would like to improve, then modify your exercise schedule accordingly. Make plans for your upcoming workout and future improvement during this time.

Your strength training or resistance training regimen might benefit from include warm-up and cool-down exercises to maximize performance, lower risk of injury, and speed up recovery. To help you achieve your long-term fitness and health goals, incorporate warm-up and cool-down exercises into your workouts on a regular basis.

Recognizing Nutrition and Recuperation

To get the most out of strength or resistance training and to support muscle growth, regeneration, and general performance, it is essential to understand recovery and nutrition. Here's how to maximize your strength training routine's diet and recuperation:

recuperation

Rest and Sleep: To encourage muscle growth and regeneration, give yourself enough time to relax and recuperate in between sessions. For the purpose of promoting healing and general health, aim for 7-9 hours of good sleep each night.

Active Recovery: Include days in your training program dedicated to low-intensity exercises like yoga, swimming, or walking. These activities encourage blood flow and muscle relaxation without putting undue strain on your body.

Hydration: Replace fluids lost through perspiration by consuming water or electrolyte-rich beverages before, during, and after your activities to stay hydrated. Maintaining performance, avoiding dehydration, and promoting recovery all depend on adequate hydration.

CHAPTER FOUR

Nutrition Timing: To assist muscle growth and repair, eat a balanced meal or snack with protein and carbohydrates within 30 to 60 minutes of finishing a workout. This will replace your glycogen levels. For the best recovery, try to maintain a carbohydrate to protein ratio of 3:1 or 4:1.

Stretching and Foam Rolling: Include stretches and foam rolls in your cool-down to ease tense muscles, increase range of motion, and aid in healing. To relieve adhesions and knots in the muscular tissue, dedicate some time to working on the sore or tight spots.

Massage treatment: To relieve soreness in your muscles, increase circulation, and promote relaxation, think about adding massage treatment to your recuperation regimen. To target certain areas of stress and aid in recovery, licensed massage therapists can employ techniques like deep tissue massage, sports massage, or myofascial release.

Temperature treatment: To reduce inflammation, ease painful muscles, and aid in recuperation, alternate between hot and cold therapeutic approaches, such as ice baths, contrast showers, or sauna sessions. Try out several temperature cures to see which ones your body responds to the best.

Food:

Protein Intake: To assist muscle growth and repair, consume a sufficient amount of protein. Divide your daily protein intake between meals and snacks by 0.8–1 grams per pound of body weight. Lean meats, poultry, fish, eggs, dairy products, legumes, and plant-based protein sources are all excellent sources of protein.

Consumption of carbs: Consume carbs before and after your workout to fuel your exercise and restore your body's glycogen stores. For long-lasting energy and peak performance, choose complex carbs found in whole grains, fruits, vegetables, and legumes.

Good Fats: Include good fats in your diet to promote hormone production and general wellness. Incorporate monounsaturated and polyunsaturated fat sources into your meals and snacks, such as avocados, nuts, seeds, olive oil, and fatty seafood.

Hydration: To stay hydrated and support your best workout performance, sip lots of water throughout the day. Try to consume 8 to 10 glasses of water or more if you perspire a lot when exercising or in hot conditions.

Micronutrients: Eat a varied and balanced diet full of fruits, vegetables, whole grains, lean proteins, and healthy fats to make sure you're getting all the vitamins and minerals your body needs. Think about including nutrient-dense foods in your meals and snacks, such as leafy greens, vibrant fruits and vegetables, nuts, seeds, and whole grains.

Meal Timing: To keep blood sugar levels stable and supply a consistent energy source for your workouts, space out your meals and snacks appropriately throughout the day. To promote energy levels and healing, try to have a balanced meal or snack every three to four hours that consists of carbs, protein, and healthy fats.

Supplementation: If you struggle to achieve your nutritional needs through food alone, or if you have specific deficiencies, you may want to think about supplementing your diet with vitamins, minerals, or other nutrients. Before beginning any supplement regimen, speak with a medical practitioner or certified dietician to be sure the supplements are safe and suitable for your particular needs.

Incorporating recovery and nutrition as top priorities into your strength and resistance training regimen will help you gain muscle, improve your performance, and take better care of your body overall. Try a variety of recovery techniques and dietary approaches to see what suits your body and objectives the best. Then, based on your results and input, make any necessary adjustments. Always keep in mind that consistency is crucial, so make recovery and nutrition top priorities in your training program.

SUMMARY

Beginning resistance or strength training is a life-changing experience with many psychological and physical advantages. It is important that you approach this journey with patience, devotion, and a desire to develop and learn as you set out on it. As you start your strength training or resistance training adventure, keep the following points in mind:

Establish Achievable targets: To help you stay motivated and to direct your exercise, clearly define your fitness objectives and set attainable targets.

Acquire Correct Form and Technique: To increase efficiency and lower the chance of injury, concentrate on acquiring correct form and technique for every activity.

Start Gradually: As you advance, progressively up the difficulty and intensity of your exercises from starting with small weights or resistance levels.

Incorporate Variety: To keep your workouts interesting, fun, and productive, mix up your exercises, training modalities, and workout forms.

Make healing Your Top Priority: To promote muscle growth, repair, and general healing, give yourself enough time to rest and recuperate in between sessions.

Emphasis on Nutrition: To boost energy levels, performance, and recuperation, feed your body with a balanced diet full of protein, carbs, healthy fats, vitamins, and minerals.

Listen to Your Body: Pay attention to the cues your body gives you, and modify your diet, training regimen, and recuperation techniques as necessary to suit your unique requirements and objectives.

Remain Consistent: Strength training advancement requires consistency. Even on the days you don't feel inspired, follow your training plan, and acknowledge your progress as you go.

You can increase your strength, enhance your fitness, and realize your full potential by adhering to these concepts and implementing them into your strength training or resistance training program. Keep in mind that each person's journey is different, so practice self-compassion, remain dedicated to your objectives, and relish the learning and development process. You will reap the many benefits of strength training and see amazing results if you put in the necessary time and effort.

THE END